Neuropathy and Myopathy in Treated Thyroid Disease

Hypothyroid and Hyperthyoid Nerve Pain and Muscle Weakness

By: James M. Lowrance © 2011

INTRODUCTION:

Thyroid disease patients can experience a number of different complications as a result of their hypothyroid (underactive thyroid) or hyperthyroid (overactive thyroid) conditions. Two of these complications are nerve pain and dysfunction, referred to as "peripheral neuropathy" and muscle weakness with possible atrophy (shrinkage of muscles), referred to as "thyroid myopathy".

In some cases, these two problems that are co-morbid to thyroid disorders can coexist, so that they are occurring at the same time and this may be referred to as "neuromuscular disease".

This is a symptom-aspect that has less information available on it via online medical search, than do the more common thyroid-related problems, such as weight gain, joint pain and fatigue.

Within the chapters of this book, that follow, I hope to present to the reader, a general understanding of these often debilitating and potentially very serious manifestations of thyroid disease, affecting the nerves and muscles of the body, including the treatments available for them.

I present this information to you as a fellow hypothyroid patient with autoimmune thyroiditis and co-morbid peripheral neuropathy and myopathy, which inspired me to search and research the information contained in the chapters.

-Jim Lowrance

TABLE OF CONTENTS:

CHAPTER ONE

What Components of Thyroid Disease causes Neuropathy and/or Myopathy?

After reading much of the medical research that is available regarding peripheral neuropathy and myopathy that results from thyroid disease, I have come to the conclusion that these problems can potentially result from the autoimmune aspect of thyroid disease or from the metabolic aspect of it or as a result of both these components, simultaneously.

While myopathy is simply a term for muscle weakness that can include atrophy (muscle wasting), peripheral neuropathy is a term that includes sensory symptoms (i.e. burning, tingling and numbness), motor symptoms (i.e. muscle weakness and difficulty controlling movements in them) and autonomic symptoms (i.e. changes in involuntary body functions, such as digestion, sweating, cardiopulmonary and other organ functions). In some patients with nerve pain, only one limb or area of their body is affected (mono-neuropathy).

Others see many areas of the body affected simultaneously (poly-neuropathy).

Autoimmune Hypothyroidism

The autoimmune aspect of thyroid disease that can be involved in the previously-described symptoms and others is the disease process that results in hormone imbalances of either the underactive or overactive thyroid types. The underactive type, also referred to as "hypothyroidism", is often the result of auto-antibodies from the immune system, that mistakenly attack the thyroid gland, which is referred to as autoimmune thyroiditis.

The types of hypothyroid autoimmunity are somewhat varied but the most common type in industrialized countries is "Hashimoto's disease", also referred to as "chronic lymphocytic thyroiditis". This common form of thyroiditis, results from the creation of auto-antibodies, from the immune system, that attack key thyroid proteins.

7

These proteins are responsible for the manufacture of thyroid hormones, from iodine that enters the body via the diet.

These two key proteins are the "thyroid Peroxidase" and the "thyroglobulin" and when these are attacked and destroyed by auto-antibodies, they are referred to as the "anti-thyroidperoxidase" and "anti-thyroglobulin" antibodies (abbreviated on blood lab tests as "Anti-TPO" and anti-TG").

These eventually cause enough damage and destruction to the thyroid gland as to cause it to manufacture abnormally low levels of thyroid hormone, which reduces the speed of metabolism in the body. The purpose of these hormones is to regulate a proper level of metabolism -- the production of energy that results from things consumed into the body (i.e. food, water and oxygen).

Autoimmune Hyperthyroidism

In the case of autoimmune overactive thyroid gland disease, also referred to as "Graves' disease", the type of auto-antibodies that cause the opposite effect of abnormally high thyroid antibodies in the body, are called "thyroid stimulating immunoglobulin" (abbreviated "TSI"). These are sent from the immune system and attach to key proteins in the thyroid gland, causing them to become overly-stimulated in producing thyroid hormone from iodine.

Some medical sources state that the TSI antibody mimics the effects of a naturally occurring hormone sent from the pituitary brain-gland, called "thyroid stimulating hormone" (abbreviated "TSH"). The pituitary gland fluctuates in the level of this necessary hormone that it sends to the thyroid gland, to properly regulate the amount of thyroid hormones manufactured and dispersed throughout all the cells of the body.

It does-so, by sensing how much of these hormones the body needs at any given time, the main ones being the "T4" (containing 4 iodine molecules) and the "T3" (containing 3 iodine molecules). It is a very sensitive system that adjusts to physical activity levels and other factors that require changes in bodily metabolism but it becomes disrupted when the thyroid gland is being attacked by either hypothyroid or hyperthyroid causing antibodies.

Autoimmunity of any kind is a strange thing. With autoimmune diseases, the body begins to attack itself for reasons that we simply have no understanding of at this stage; this despite there being significant numbers of medical research studies on the subject that have been published by medical groups for decades. For some reason, the immune system will begin to attack natural, normal tissues in the body, as if they are something that presents a danger to the rest of the body. These specially-created antibodies are usually sent-out to destroy viruses and bacteria or to control allergens that might enter the body.

Neuropathy and Myopathy in Treated Thyroid Disease

These offending cells are contracted into the body via airborne particles that are breathed-in or that are consumed in food or water. When a part of the body that does not present a threat to us is attacked by this autoimmune response, apart from these obvious reasons, it is a mystery to medical doctors and researchers who diagnose and study diseases of autoimmunity.

Bodily Metabolism Depends on Thyroid Hormones

Since both the muscles and nerves are highly dependent upon a normal metabolism to operate correctly, they can become negatively hindered and possibly damaged by thyroid hormone imbalances that are severe or when treatment is delayed for them.

My belief after corresponding with literally 100s of fellow-thyroid patients since the year 2003 is that some patients experience problems with neuropathy and/or myopathy, even after receiving adequate or optimal thyroid treatment and I am in-fact one of them.

The "metabolic aspect" of thyroid disease previously described which causes either a slowed hypothyroid metabolism or a sped-up hyperthyroid metabolism can be a factor that causes development of neuropathy and myopathy as well. This is true even if it is secondarily-caused, rather than being a problem within the thyroid gland itself.

Secondary causes of thyroid dysfunction result from other problems within the body, that affect thyroid hormone production but that still affect bodily metabolism as a result, due to an imbalance in the hormones. If the pituitary gland for example, becomes disrupted due to a tumor that develops within it, this can cause it to either slow-down or speed-up the dispersing of TSH to the thyroid gland. This is referred to as "central hypothyroidism" and "central hyperthyroidism", meaning there is a problem occurring in the brain-center from which proper thyroid regulation normally originates. In females, tumors on the ovaries can be a secondary cause of an overactive thyroid gland as well.

Neuropathy and Myopathy in Treated Thyroid Disease

Small tumors within the thyroid gland itself, called "hot nodules" which would actually be a "primary cause" of hyperthyroidism but that can occur without thyroid autoimmunity being present, can also develop. A long-term, uncorrected abnormal increase or decrease in metabolism due to thyroid hormone imbalances can become detrimental to the body.

Symptoms of Thyroid Hormone Disorders

When hypothyroidism occurs due to any cause, the resulting symptoms can include the following.

• Muscle and joint aches
• Nerve pain in the extremities

• Feeling cold in warm temperatures

• Dry skin and brittle fingernails

• Hair that has become brittle and breaks off or falls out

• Thinning of the eyebrows and loss of the outer 1/3 portion of them

Neuropathy and Myopathy in Treated Thyroid Disease

- Unexplained weight gain with no diet change

- Constipation

- Slowed heart rate and breathing

- Depression

- Physical tiredness/fatigue
- Myxedema (fluid retention-tissue swelling)

- Feeling a fullness or tightness in the throat (goiter)

When hyperthyroidism occurs due to any cause, the resulting symptoms can include the following.

- Muscle and joint aches aches (possible muscle atrophy)
- Nerve pain in the extremities
- Rapid heart rate
- Hyperventilation
- Hypertension
- Sweating
- Inability to sleep
- Nervousness and anxiety
- Diarrhea ...

Neuropathy and Myopathy in Treated Thyroid Disease

...

- Excessive energy followed by fatigue
- Hair loss
- Weight loss
- Osteoporosis (bone loss)
- Myxedema
- Swelling of the thyroid gland (goiter)

In many cases the "myxedema" symptom, shown in both lists, is directly related to nerve pain in the body due to fluid-retention causing excessive pressure on the nerves.

When either of these thyroid hormone imbalances has been diagnosed, treatment for them will begin. In the chapter that follows, diagnoses methods and treatments will be discussed.

Neuropathy and Myopathy in Treated Thyroid Disease

CHAPTER TWO

Treatments for Hypothyroid and Hyperthyroid Hormone Imbalances

For both hypothyroid and hyperthyroid disorders, blood lab testing is often the type of diagnostic method that first detects them. A panel is often ordered when symptoms indicate a thyroid hormone imbalance is present and it will often consist of the T4, T3 and TSH levels.

If additional labs are ordered, these will usually be imaging tests, such as radioactive iodine uptake scans, thyroid ultrasound, MRI, CAT scans and occasionally, a fine-needle tissue biopsy is extracted from the thyroid gland for analysis.

The Sensitivity of TSH Blood Testing

If a thyroid condition is not suspected and a patient is simply having a battery of tests ordered for a routine medical evaluation, the only test that might be included to evaluate thyroid function will be the TSH.

This test is often the most sensitive for detecting a lowering or increasing T4 and/or T3 level. The reason for this being, that TSH is increased to abnormally high levels, to maintain proper thyroid hormone levels when they are decreased even slightly, due to a diseased thyroid gland or due to a secondary cause resulting in hypothyroidism.

If the gland has begun to produce too-much thyroid hormone due to primary or secondary hyperthyroidism the opposite will occur and the TSH will begin to drop to below-normal levels, even early into the thyroid over-activity. During this process, the pituitary gland may be able to correct the T4 and T3 for a period of time but it struggles to do so and eventually the thyroid hormones also become imbalanced, as the TSH fails to maintain them at normal values.

Many patients' thyroid disorders first manifest with an abnormal TSH and the T4 and T3 will remain temporarily-normal at this juncture. This is referred-to as "subclinical thyroid disorder".

For many patients; their condition will stay at a subclinical stage for months or even years.

If a patient experiences symptoms of either overactive or underactive thyroid glands, even when only the TSH is abnormal, some doctors will begin treatment at this stage. If symptoms are not present with an abnormal TSH level, a doctor might instead retest the patients' blood level of TSH, every few months to see if the disorder is progressing to an overt level (full blown).

When Do Doctors Start Treatment for Thyroid Disorders?

Different thyroid-specializing doctors use a different standard for determining when to treat developing hypothyroid and hyperthyroid disorders. Some doctors will treat hypothyroid patients whose TSH is elevated but whose T4 and T3 levels are normal, as long as TSH reaches a level of at-least "10.0" or higher (the highest normal value at labs, currently averages about "5.0").

Some doctors will also treat hypothyroid patients if both the TSH is elevated and the T4 or T3 are below normal on blood test results. Yet other doctors factor-in the presence or absence of symptoms, as previously mentioned.

The same type logic is used by some doctors in regard to hyperthyroid conditions as well but in this case, the TSH lowest normal value averages approximately "0.3" at testing labs, currently. If a hyperthyroid patient has indications of an overactive metabolism (symptoms), with a below-normal TSH but their T4 and T3 remain within normal values, the doctor may opt to start them on treatment as well and most doctors will certainly do-so if both TSH is abnormally low and the T4 and/or T3 are abnormally high.

Types of Thyroid Disease Treatments

Hypothyroidism treatment is relatively simple compared to treatments for hyperthyroidism and consists of simply supplementing the hypothyroid patient with a daily dose of T4 or combination T4 and T3 hormone replacement medication.

The prescribed dose will correct the low thyroid hormone levels over time but this might take a process of several months, with the dose starting at a minimal level and being titrated upward (adjusted by gradual increases), until the patients' TSH, T4 and T3 levels return to adequate or optimal normal values. This is determined via repeat blood testing, every few weeks or months.

Hyperthyroidism treatments are slightly more complicated and varied, depending on the cause of the overactive thyroid gland and the severity of it. In some cases, a patient will only require the prescribing of an "anti-thyroid drug", which slows the production of thyroid hormones, returning thyroid function to a normal level.

Other patients might need a beta-blocker medication prescribed, which will correct hypertension and tachycardia (rapid heart rate) if these are present and if an anti-thyroid drug alone does not correct them. A combination of both type drugs can in some cases, correct the hyperthyroidism symptoms more adequately.

Neuropathy and Myopathy in Treated Thyroid Disease

Some hyperthyroid patients need corrective surgeries, to move part or all of their thyroid glands (partial or total thyroidectomy) or they will be referred for radioactive iodine ablation of the gland. This latter mentioned procedure, abbreviated "RAI" is performed by a qualified doctor who administers a dose of radioactive iodine to a patient, which is immediately absorbed by the gland and causes destruction of all tissues within it, so that it is basically dissolved/removed from the body within several weeks following the treatment.

Many doctors are now seeing more value in surgical removal because this often assures that the diseased thyroid tissue is fully removed. Thyroidectomy also becomes necessary in cases of thyroid cancer or when hot nodules are present but in the case of non-malignant nodules, only partial removal may become necessary.

Once thyroid removal of either type has been completed, the patient will require thyroid hormone replacement therapy.

Neuropathy and Myopathy in Treated Thyroid Disease

Treatment is similar to that of hypothyroid patients, due to their thyroid glands not being fully present or not present at all, to supply thyroid hormone for proper bodily metabolism.

Is Prescribed Thyroid Hormone Always Adequate?

While these treatments correct thyroid hormone imbalances, some patients may still go on to see progression of neuropathy or myopathy symptoms. As stated earlier, my belief is that the "autoimmune" aspect of thyroid diseases may be responsible for this or it is also possible that supplemented thyroid hormones do not nourish the body and its metabolism as well as do naturally-occurring thyroid hormones.

This second possibility is certainly a theory at this point however, even the pharmaceutical companies who manufacture synthetic and natural brands of prescribed thyroid hormones, claim that certain competing brands do not as adequately resolve the complications of hypothyroid conditions.

Inadequacies in some manufactured hormones have actually resulted in the FDA requiring recalls of certain types, after dosage-inconsistency were found in them (pharmacies required to take the product off-sale). Even the major brand manufacturers have been affected by these recalls in past years.

CHAPTER THREE

Why Thyroid Treatments may not Resolve Neuropathy and Myopathy Symptoms

There are a number of reason why thyroid disease treatments might not fully resolve cases of peripheral neuropathy or thyroid myopathy. As mentioned in the previous chapter, one reason could be that thyroid hormones coming into the body from the outside (prescribed), rather than from the thyroid gland, naturally, may be less adequate.

As also previously mentioned, thyroid hormone replacement is not just required by hypothyroid patients but also by hyperthyroid patients who have had thyroidectomies or radioactive iodine ablations performed on them.

Undertreated Hypothyroid Patients

Some doctors, who are less-qualified to administer thyroid hormone replacement therapy, may also have a tendency to under-treat some patients.

Neuropathy and Myopathy in Treated Thyroid Disease

This can be due to the concern some doctors have for inducing thyrotoxicity (over-treatment causing hyperthyroidism) and as a result, they are reluctant to optimize treatment for patients to prevent the risk of inducing hyperthyroid symptoms. Under-treated patients carry the risk of complications from what amounts to being kept in a subclinical hypothyroid state by their doctors, including those affecting nerves and muscles.

Once Damage has been Done

I also believe that it's entirely possible that once nerve or muscle damage has occurred in thyroid patients, whether from hyperthyroid or hypothyroid conditions, the treatments they receive may not stop progression of further damage or the preceding damage is not fully reversible.

Medical sources that inform the public about "Thyroid Myopathy", state that the disease can be progressive, similar to types of muscular dystrophy.

Neuropathy and Myopathy in Treated Thyroid Disease

Once reaching this level, it then becomes a disease entity of itself. Once this occurs, treatments are designed to address symptoms and to comfort patients as much as possible, rather than to reverse the disease process, if it has been established that it is irreversible.

Sensory, Autonomic and Motor Nerves

This same applies to some cases of peripheral neuropathy (PN), which once damaging the nerves, continues to cause sensory symptoms, such as burning, tingling and stabbing pains to the extremities via the "sensory nerves" and that can progress to the trunk of the body and to the nerves that regulate involuntary organ functions as well (autonomic neuropathy).

If the "motor nerves" are also affected by a case of PN (those that affect muscle strength and movement), this may in some cases be placed into the category of a neuromuscular disease.

This is not common and is more likely to occur in thyroid patients with other autoimmune diseases (i.e. Lupus, Rheumatoid Arthritis, Celiac disease and Sjogren 's syndrome) and in those with co-morbid diabetes than in those with thyroid disease only.

In my personal case however, I have had other autoimmune diseases and diabetes ruled-out repeatedly but I continue to experience neuropathy and myopathy symptoms, even after more than eight years of hypothyroid treatment, that has been optimized best-possible.

Research Regarding Neuropathy and Myopathy in Treated Thyroid Patients

Following are quotes from the U.S. National Institutes of Health (PubMed), regarding unresolved neuropathy and myopathy in treated hypothyroid patients, from five different research studies.

1.Pain and small-fiber neuropathy in patients with hypothyroidism (U.S. National Library of Medicine - PubMed) ---

"Conclusions: Some patients treated for hypothyroidism have symptoms and findings compatible with small-fiber neuropathy or "hyper phenomena" indicating central sensitization. ...of Eighteen patients...Eight were classified as having large fiber neuropathy..."

2.Hypothyroidism and polyneuropathy. (U.S. National Library of Medicine - PubMed) ---

"Using standard electrophysiological criteria, a definite diagnosis of polyneuropathy was made in 28 cases (72%). The commonest sites of abnormal nerve conduction were the sensory nerves, especially the sural nerve."

3.Hypothyroid neuropathy and myopathy: clinical and electrodiagnostic longitudinal findings. (U.S. National Library of Medicine - PubMed) ---

"This case shows that thyroid hormone replacement eliminates the neuropathic manifestations of severe hypothyroidism.

In contrast, the myopathic features, such as weakness and muscle wasting, may persist despite maintenance of the euthyroid state."

4.Neuromuscular status of thyroid diseases: a prospective clinical and electrodiagnostic study. (U.S. National Library of Medicine - PubMed) ---

Among the thyroid patients, 17 (42.5%) patients were diagnosed with mononeuropathy and polyneuropathy. Entrapment neuropathy was observed in 30% and diffuse neuropathy in 10% of the patients. Myopathy findings were observed in 2 patients.

5.Aspects of peripheral nerve involvement in patients with treated hypothyroidism. (U.S. National Library of Medicine - PubMed) ---

"RESULTS: Sixty-three per cent of the patients with 'pure' hypothyroidism had abnormalities on NCS, 25% had reduced IENF density and 31% had abnormalities on QST.

Four patients (25%) met criteria for small fibre polyneuropathy, the other (75%) were classified as having mixed fiber polyneuropathy.

I believe this research makes the point very clear, that not all thyroid patients see recovery from neuropathy or myopathy symptoms, following proper treatment.

Co-morbid Nutritional Deficiencies

A final reason for treated thyroid patients continuing to experience neuropathy and/or myopathy symptoms or actually developing them in spite of being treated, that I will also mention, are "nutritional deficiencies" occurring co-morbid to thyroid disease.

All nutrients, which include vitamins, minerals and electrolytes, have potential to negatively affect nerve and/or muscle function when they become imbalanced and this can be true whether they become deficient or abnormally elevated in the body.

Common deficiencies that are found in thyroid patients include vitamins B12 and D and the mineral-electrolyte deficiencies potassium and magnesium. Others can potentially occur as well however, including deficiencies in other B-vitamins, as well as vitamin E and other types of essential nutrients.

When myopathy and/or neuropathy are occurring in spite of adequate thyroid treatment, a full nutritional blood panel should be ordered. All nutritional deficiencies are treatable and corrective supplementation of nutrients can correct problems in the nerves and muscles that are dependent upon normal levels of them.

Hyperthyroid patients are at risk for developing nutritional deficiencies, due to their sped-up digestion, which causes food to pass through them very quickly. Most patients experience ongoing diarrhea and this can result in malabsorption of essential nutrients over time. Once their hyperthyroidism is corrected, they may still need low nutrients replaced via proper supplementation (doctor-approved).

Neuropathy and Myopathy in Treated Thyroid Disease

My Own Diagnosis of Thyroid Disease and Deficient Nutrients

My case of Hashimoto's thyroiditis, diagnosed in year-2003 has not been passed down to me from previous generations. Neither my parents, grandparents nor even my great grandparents were known to have autoimmune thyroid disease of any kind. Some medical research, as stated by the AACE (American Association of Endocrinologist), states that thyroid autoimmunity is inherited in approximately 50% of cases that are diagnosed. In my case it is not inherited and my belief is that EBV (the "Epstein - Barr virus" -- that causes mononucleosis) is very possibly a direct cause of my autoimmune hypothyroidism. The correlations to contracting the virus in my childhood and to my ongoing immune system problems, from that point forward, are simply too striking to be coincidental.

When I was approximately age-10, I became very ill with mononucleosis and I was out of school with the virus for over 6 weeks.

Neuropathy and Myopathy in Treated Thyroid Disease

My two brothers and my sister never manifested any symptoms of mono, in spite of being in close contact with me during my bout with the illness. Once the viral illnesses had run its course, the glands in my neck returned to normal size, my fever resolved and my fatigue improved. I returned to school and normal activities but my body continued to manifest problems that I now know were related to dysfunction of my immune system. I developed childhood asthma and I experienced colds and viruses, more frequently than did my siblings. I remember on one occasion, my family contracted a respiratory virus and upon all of us our seeing a doctor on the same day, he informed my parents that my case was the most severe.

I mention this regarding EBV, due to the fact that many medical research studies have been published, linking EBV to the development of neurological conditions. This gives me yet one other possibility of a cause for both my thyroid autoimmunity and my co-morbid neuropathy symptoms.

My belief is that autoimmune thyroid diseases are among the common post-viral effects of EBV. I noticed sometime ago, that an Oklahoma-based medical research group, was attempting to patent a vaccination for EBV and in their statements included on their patent application, they cite the fact that the virus has been implemented as a cause of many different autoimmune diseases. My feeling is that the immune system is adamant about eradicating the body of this virus. When it cannot do-so completely, it may begin to attack major organs or hormone glands that contain the virus, including a person's thyroid gland. This is a theory at this point but one I feel has real merit in light of medical research studies.

My Treatment since Year 2003

In my case as a hypothyroid patient, treated since 2003, with ongoing nerve and muscle symptoms, I was found to be deficient in vitamins D and E and I was found to have insufficient levels of B12 as well (low-normal).

My blood electrolyte level of potassium was found to be slightly below normal and my phosphate became slightly elevated, however, the phosphate normalized with replacing the low vitamin levels, while the potassium required supplementation and diet changes to correct.

Some thyroid patients can benefit from a good daily multivitamin and they can certainly benefit from modifying their diets to include more fruits, vegetables, nuts and grains versus simple carbohydrates which come in the form of junk foods. Regular exercise helps nutrients and hormones to circulate better in the body and helps the body to rid itself of toxins and extra fat that can block some of the positive effects of nutrients.

CHAPTER FOUR

Considering all Treatment Options for Thyroid Neuropathy and Myopathy

Neuropathy and myopathy in thyroid disease patients can be improved in most cases to varied degrees as previously discussed. For some patients, these problems may completely resolve over time, while others may still experience them.

The first consideration in resolving these symptoms best-possible is to make sure thyroid hormone therapies are optimized, best possible. For some thyroid doctors, this means getting the TSH level suppressed into the low-normal or even the lowest-normal value and getting the T4 and T3 levels raised to above mid-range and possibly up to highest-normal values. Needs are varied among different patients and this is why it is important that a qualified doctor is sought for treatment and one who considers each patients' symptoms as well, rather than basing treatment on blood lab values alone.

Neuropathy and Myopathy in Treated Thyroid Disease

Getting tested for possible nutritional deficiencies can also be very important as previously mentioned, especially if thyroid hormone correction does not adequately relieve muscle and nerve related symptoms.

Drugs that Treat Nerve and/or Muscle Pain

There are many types of medications, including both the prescribed types and those that can be purchased over-the-counter to help regulate pain involving nerves and/or muscles. There are however three classes of drugs that are specifically directed at relieving pain in-general, which include the following types and brands.

• **Over-The-Counter Drugs:**
• Acetaminophen
• Aspirin
• ibuprofen
• Naproxen

- **Antidepressants:**

- Tricyclic Antidepressants (TCA's) – (i.e. Types: Amitriptyline and Nortriptiline)

- Selective Serotonin Reuptake Inhibitors (SSRI) – (i.e. Brands: Paxil, Prozac, Zoloft)

- **Anticonvulsants:**

- Gabapentin

- Carbamazepine

- Felbamate

- Valproic Acid

- Clonazepam

- Phenytoin

In severe cases of pain, that fails to improve with medication, patients may be referred for "nerve block treatments", which consist of a series of injections into the areas of pain, using a substance such as alcohol or phenol (carbolic acid) to interrupt pain signals. The injections are given at regular intervals, to help with ongoing, severe pain.

Neuropathy and Myopathy in Treated Thyroid Disease

Nerve Entrapment Therapies

When pain is referred from a nerve that is being pinched (nerve entrapment), treatments will be directed at relieving the pressure on the affected nerves. Some nerve entrapments cause significant pain, such as those affecting the "sciatic nerve" (a large nerve that runs from the back, into the legs and feet), the "median nerve" (affecting the wrists and hands) and the posterior tibial nerve (affecting the feet and toes).

Treatments may include surgical procedures, massage and chiropractic therapies, temperature applications (ice packs or heating pads) and isolation, meaning a period of restricted or non-movement of limbs or other body-parts that contain entrapped nerves (movement may be encouraged if muscles are primarily affected). In some cases, nerve-stimulation devices are used in attempt to stimulate proper impulses from nerves that have been affected by long-term entrapment.

It is important to see a qualified medical doctor for the evaluation and treatment of thyroid disorders and for referral to treatments for co-morbid problems affecting the nerves and/or muscles, when thyroid treatment alone does not resolve them. I offer my most sincere "best wishes" to the readers of this book, who are seeking treatment-solutions for their thyroid-related myopathies and neuropathies.

(END) --*See the bonus chapter following below, for a little humor (very little).*

CHAPTER FIVE

Eight Thyroid Disease Knock-Knock Jokes: (Laughing at the Expense of the Metabolic Butterfly)

Some readers might think "What! – A thyroid disease joke chapter – you've got to be kidding!" and I would respond by saying "Yes, I am kidding and that's the purpose of this chapter!" We're doing something that comedy often does, by taking a serious subject and finding a way to laugh about it. Why not?!

As thyroid patients who go through the ups and downs of our diseases, why shouldn't we find a way to derive some humor from it? I believe by doing so, that we can actually find better coping as we may sometimes struggle with the fact that we're living with a lifelong disease that will require ongoing treatment for most of us, as we live-out our lives in this world.

Neuropathy and Myopathy in Treated Thyroid Disease

What better way is there, to take some of the seriousness out of the fear we sometimes experience when we're having a flare of symptoms or we're experiencing some emotional phases with our diseases, than to find ways to laugh about it?

It is my sincere hope that fellow-patients or anyone who enjoys a good laugh will do-so, while reading this added bonus-chapter.

As a patient with autoimmune thyroiditis that is causing me lifelong hypothyroidism and co morbid health problems, plus a need for daily treatments for it, I feel that laughter truly is a good medicine that can help me to cope better, when I'm feeling a bit down due to my disease and its symptoms. I hope this proves to be the case for those who read this chapter as well!

While some of these knock-knock jokes are a bit on the corny side (some smack in the middle of it), I think they will still get you to smile a little and hopefully some of them will get a few genuine giggles out of you.

Neuropathy and Myopathy in Treated Thyroid Disease

So, with the boring chapter-introduction out of the way, let's get to the comedy.

Knock-knock

Who's there?

I Goiter

I goiter who?

I goiter go to the doctor, cause my neck feels swollen.

Knock-knock

Who's there?

R.U. Goins

R.U. Goins who?

R.U. Goins to the doctor, cause your mood seems like it's hypothyroid.

Neuropathy and Myopathy in Treated Thyroid Disease

Knock-knock

Who's there?

I.M. Crabbie

I.M. Crabbie who?

I.M. crabbie because I forgot to take my thyroid pill this morning.

Knock-knock

Who's there?

B.A. Angel

B.A. Angel who?

B.A. angel and order me a double cheeseburger, my hypothyroidism is making me hungry.

Knock-knock

Who's there?

B4 U

Neuropathy and Myopathy in Treated Thyroid Disease

B4 U Who?

B4 U call me a zombie, remember that I might be having brain fog.

Knock-knock

Who's there?

I.R. Moody

I.R. Moody who?

I.R. Moody today, so don't push your luck by pushing my buttons.

Knock-knock

Who's there?

I.B. Shedding

I.B. Shedding who?

Neuropathy and Myopathy in Treated Thyroid Disease

I.B. Shedding hair, so don't mistake my pillow for a raccoon in the bed.

Knock-knock

Who's there?

M.I. Goen

M.I. Goen who?

M.I. goen to the doctor soon, cause my thyroid hormone pills don't seem to be working?

Neuropathy and Myopathy in Treated Thyroid Disease

About the Author:

I am a husband, father, grandfather and lifetime contract salesman, with experience in health writing that began in 2004. I completed theological studies with Liberty University in 1996. I formerly served as editor and forum moderator of Thyroid Health for a major multi-topic content site and as a general health writer for another, on which I achieved Editor's Choice Awards for my articles on health subjects.

In 2003 I was diagnosed with hypothyroidism; "Hashimoto's thyroiditis" being the cause. This autoimmune form of thyroid disease that causes destruction of the thyroid gland resulted in my also developing "Chronic Fatigue Syndrome", due to a compromised immune system with severe co-morbid "Adrenal Fatigue". I also suffered severe anxiety symptoms, including panic attacks early into the onset of Hashimoto's thyroiditis (Hashitoxicosis). I was aso diagnosed with peripheral neuropathy and thyroid myopathy, with co-morbid nutritional deficiencies.

My eventual receiving of diagnoses was a difficult process with proper diagnostic testing not being ordered by the first doctors I sought treatment from.

These types of issues were inspiration for me to become proactive in my own health care and to self-educate myself on these health disorders, which I have done extensively since 2003. I now enjoy sharing this information with other patients experiencing my same health disorders.

(END)